AF505145

Copyright ©2020 ARNOLD KUNTZ PH.D

CONTENTS

INTRODUCTION

Whether your pain is from arthritis, cancer treatments, fibromyalgia, or an old injury, you need to find a way to get your pain under control. What's the best approach to do that?

The first step in pain management is scheduling an appointment with your doctor to determine the cause of your pain and learn which pain management approach is often the most effective for it. There are many different pain management options available: You can find the right treatment combination to get the relief you need.

Pain is an unpleasant sensory and emotional experience. I think that's extraordinarily important. When we focus only on the sensory aspect, we fail to appreciate the suffering component of the pain, which is important to recognize because pain is not what occurs at the periphery.

WHAT IS PAIN?

If you've ever touched a hot stove, you know pain. Pain is a signal from our body that something is not right. Pain receptors in our bodies send electrical messages to the spinal cord and brain, which we interpret as pain. In certain situations, you are able to retract from pain to stop the hurt. In most cases, however, the pain is either short-lived (acute) or ongoing (chronic).

Medically, pain can be a signal for another condition. It can be due to a physical injury, a malignant disease, or an emotional upset. Most types of physical pain can be treated with pain relievers, but it's important to use these safely. What kinds of pain medications are there? Analgesics such as acetaminophen or paracetamol are used to treat mild or moderate pain, and can also be used to reduce temperature in fevers. Narcotic analgesics such as codeine can be used alone or in combination with other analgesics for stronger pain, such as dental pain, menstrual pain or migraines. Short-term use of these medication is important. Non-steroidal anti-inflammatory drugs (including aspirin) are used to reduce pain associated with inflammation, such as sports injuries, and can also be used to relieve fever.

Acetaminophen, the NSAIDs ibuprofen or naproxen, and aspirin are all available over-the-counter (OTC).

ARNOLD KUNTZ PH.D

Pain results from a variety of pathological processes. It is expressed differently by each patient depending on cultural background, age, etc. It is a subjective experience meaning that only the individual is able to assess his/her level of pain. Regular assessment of the intensity of pain is indispensable in establishing effective treatment.

COMMON PAIN CONDITIONS

There are many acute and chronic pain conditions, including:

Musculoskeletal Pain

Back and leg pain

Neck, shoulder and arm pain

"Whiplash" injuries

Motor vehicle, work-related and sport injuries

Post-surgical pain

Arthritis

Fibromyalgia

Cancer Pain

Primary and metastatic cancer pain (cancer that has spread to distant areas of the body)

Medication side effect management

PAIN LINKED TO OTHER CONDITIONS

Vascular pain

Raynaud's Disease

Psychogenic Pain

Trigeminal neuralgia

Spinal cord injury

Spasticity

Pelvic pain

Pediatric pain

Neuropathic Pain

Complex Regional Pain Syndrome (RSD)

Shingles

Neuralgia

Nerve Injuries

Phantom limb pain

Over-the-Counter (OTC) Pain Medications

Acetaminophen (Tylenol)

Ibuprofen (Advil, Motrin)

Naproxen (Aleve)

Aspirin (Bayer)

Over-the-counter medications, which you can buy without a prescription, are good for many types of pain.

Acetaminophen

Acetaminophen (Tylenol) is good for relieving minor pain, headache and fever. It is less irritating to the stomach than other over-the-counter pain medications, such as NSAIDs. It can, however, be toxic to the liver if you take more than the recommended dose.

Be sure to look at the total amount oacetaminophen in all of the medications you take and do not exceed 4 grams (4,000 mg) of acetaminophen per day in adults. Also avoid excess alcohol consumption if you take acetaminophen to lower further risk of liver toxicity.

NSAIDs

Aspirin, naproxen (Aleve), and ibuprofen (Advil, Motrin) are examples of non-steroidal anti-inflammatory drugs (NSAIDs). These reduce inflammation caused by injury, arthritis, or fever. NSAIDs also relieve pain associated with menstruation, dental pain, and headache. Take these medications in regular dosing intervals as directed by the manufacturer on the package. If you have high blood pressure, kidney disease, or a history of gastrointestinal ulcers or bleeding, you should consult your health care provider before using any over-the-counter NSAID.

NSAIDs can increase your risk of heart attack or stroke that can be fatal, especially if you use it long term or take high doses, or if you have heart disease. Even people without heart disease or risk factors could have a stroke or heart attack while taking NSAIDs. Do not use an NSAID just before or after heart bypass surgery (coronary artery bypass graft, or CABG). Talk to your doctor about the use of over-the-counter NSAIDs.

CAN YOU GIVE ASPIRIN TO CHILDREN?

DO NOT give aspirin to children. Reye's syndrome is associated with the use of aspirin to treat children with viral infections, such as chicken pox or the flu. This syndrome can cause brain and liver damage. Reye syndrome is most often seen in children ages 4 to 12.

PRESCRIPTION PAIN RELIEVERS

Prescription medications may be needed for more severe types of pain. There are specific uses and risks of prescription narcotic and non-narcotic medications. Because these drugs can be linked with side effects like drowsiness, constipation, slowed breathing and addiction, it is best to try non-narcotic pain relievers for mild, temporary, pain. For nerve (neuropathic) pain, anticonvulsant medications such as gabapentin may be used. There are alternate methods to help reduce pain that may be helpful instead of, or in addition to, pain medications. These include:

Heat for sore or overworked muscles

Ice applied to recent injuries (such as a sprained ankle)

MASSAGE

Resting the affected body part

Biofeedback or relaxation techniques.

Consult your doctor if pain lasts longer than a few days, if over-the-counter pain medications are not helping to reduce the pain, or if other symptoms arise. A consultation with a pain clinic or other specialist may be helpful for control of long-term pain.

CLINICAL FEATURES

Pain assessment

– Intensity: use a simple verbal scale in children over 5 years and adults, and NFCS or FLACC scales in children less than 5 years (see Pain evaluation scales).

– Pattern: sudden, intermittent, chronic; at rest, at night, on movement, during care procedures, etc.

– Character: burning, cramping, spasmodic, radiating, etc.

– Aggravating or relieving factors, etc.

CLINICAL EXAMINATION

– Of the organ or area where the pain is located.

– Specific signs of underlying disease (e.g. bone or osteoarticular pain may be caused by a vitamin C deficiency) and review of all systems.

– Associated signs (fever, weight loss, etc.).

SYNTHESIS

The synthesis of information gathered during history taking and clinical examination allows aetiological diagnosis and orients treatment. It is important to distinguish:

– Nociceptive pain: it presents most often as acute pain and the cause-effect relationship is usually obvious (e.g. acute post-operative pain, burns, trauma, renal colic, etc.). The pain may be present in different forms, but neurological exam is normal. Treatment is relatively well standardized.

– Neuropathic pain, due to a nerve lesion (section, stretching, ischaemia): most often chronic pain. On a background of constant, more or less localized pain, such as paraesthesia or burning, there are recurrent acute attacks such as electric shock-like pain, frequently associated with disordered sensation (anaesthesia, hypo or hyperaesthesia). This type of pain is linked to viral infections directly affecting the CNS (herpes simplex, herpes zoster), neural compression by tumors, post- amputation pain, paraplegia, etc.

– Mixed pain (cancer, HIV) for which management requires a broader approach.

TREATMENT

Treatment depends on the type and intensity of the pain. It may be both aetiological and symptomatic if a treatable cause is identified. Treatment is symptomatic only in other cases (no cause found, non-curable disease).

Nociceptive pain
The WHO classifies analgesics used for this type of pain on a three-step ladder:

– Step 1: non-opioid analgesics such as paracetamol and nonsteroidal anti-inflammatory drugs (NSAIDs).

– Step 2: weak opioid analgesics such as codeine and tramadol. Their combination with one or two Step 1 analgesics is recommended.

– Step 3: strong opioid analgesics, first and foremost morphine. Their combination with one or two Step 1 analgesics is recommended.

The treatment of pain is based on a few fundamental concepts:
– Pain can only be treated correctly if it is correctly evaluated. The only person who can evaluate the intensity of pain is the patient himself. The use of pain assessment scales is invaluable.

– The pain evaluation observations should be recorded in the patient chart in the same fashion as other vital signs.

– Treatment of pain should be as prompt as possible.

– It is recommended to administer analgesics in advance when appropriate (e.g. before painful care procedures).

– Analgesics should be prescribed and administered at fixed time intervals (not on demand).

– Oral forms should be used whenever possible.

– The combination of different analgesic drugs (multimodal analgesia) is advantageous.

– Start with an analgesic from the level presumed most effective: e.g., in the event of a fractured femur, start with a Step 3 analgesic.

– The treatment and dose chosen are guided by the assessment of pain intensity, but also by the patient's response which may vary significantly from one person to another.

NEUROPATHIC PAIN

Commonly used analgesics are often ineffective in treating this type of pain. Treatment of neuropathic pain is based on a combination of two centrally acting drugs:

Amitriptyline PO
Adults: 25 mg once daily at bedtime (Week 1); 50 mg once daily at bedtime (Week 2); 75 mg once daily at bedtime (as of Week 3); max.150 mg daily. Reduce the dose by half in elderly patients.

Carbamazepine PO
Adults: 200 mg once daily at bedtime (Week 1); 200 mg 2 times daily (Week 2); 200 mg 3 times daily (as of Week 3)

Given its teratogenic risk, carbamazepine should only be used in women of childbearing age when covered by effective contraception (intrauterine device or injectable progestogen). It is not recommended in pregnant women.

Mixed pain
In mixed pain with a significant component of nociceptive pain, such as in cancer or AIDS, morphine is combined with antidepressants and antiepileptics.

Chronic pain
In contrast to acute pain, medical treatment alone is not always sufficient in controlling chronic pain. A multidisciplinary approach including medical treatment,

physiotherapy, psychotherapy and nursing is often necessary to allow good pain relief and encourage patient self-management.

Co-analgesics
The combination of certain drugs may be useful or even essential in the treatment of pain: antispasmodics, muscle relaxants, anxiolytics, corticosteroids, local anesthesia, etc.

TYPES OF PAIN

Acute pain can last a moment; rarely does it become chronic pain. Chronic pain persists for long periods. It is resistant to most medical treatments and cause severe problems.

Pain Classifications
Even though the experience of pain varies from one person to the next, it is possible to categorize the different types of pain.

Nerve Pain
When nerve fibers get damaged, the result can be chronic pain. Read about the very common causes of neuropathic pain, like diabetes.

Psychogenic Pain
Depression, anxiety, and other emotional problems can cause pain- or make existing pain worse.

Musculoskeletal Pain
Musculoskeletal pain is pain that affects the muscles, ligaments and tendons, and bones. Learn about the causes, symptoms, and treatments.

Chronic Muscle Pain
Use your muscles incorrectly, too much, too little and you've got muscle pain. Learn the subtle differences of muscle injuries and pain.

Central Pain Syndrome
A stroke, multiple sclerosis, or spinal cord injuries can result in chronic pain and burning syndromes from damage to brain regions.

Complex Regional Pain Syndrome
It's a baffling, intensely painful disorder that can develop from a seemingly minor injury, yet is believed to result from high levels of nerve impulses being sent to the affected disorder.

Diabetes-Related Nerve Pain (Neuropathy)
If you have diabetes, nerve damage can be a serious complication. This nerve complication can cause severe burning pain especially at night.

Shingles Pain (Postherpetic Neuralgia)
Shingles is a painful condition that arises from varicella-zoster, the same virus that causes chickenpox. Le

Trigeminal Neuralgia
It's considered one of the most painful conditions in medicine. The face pain it causes can be treated.

SYMPTOMS & CAUSES

The feeling of physical pain can vary greatly mild, sharp, severe, and dull. Learn the symptoms for different types of pain, so you can describe them to a doctor.

CAUSES OF CHRONIC PAIN

Anything from a bad mattress to stomach ulcers can cause chronic pain. While it may begin with an injury or illness, pain can develop a psychological dimension once the physical problem heals.

Compressed Nerve (Pinched Nerve)
Pinched nerves can sometimes lead to other conditions such as peripheral neuropathy, carpal tunnel syndrome, and tennis elbow.

Hand Pain Causes
With today's increasingly active society, the number of hand problems is increasing. Hand pain has a wide variety of specific causes and treatments.

Hip Pain: Causes and Symptoms
Despite its durability, the hip joint isn't indestructible. With age and use, the cartilage can wear down or become damaged.

Causes of Neck and Shoulder Pain
Neck and shoulder pain can be classified in many different ways. Learn how they are diagnosed and treated.

Chronic Knee and Joint Pain
Arthritis that affects your "shock absorbers" is the cause of

pain and disability in knee and hip joints that can lead to surgery.

Whiplash

A car accident or any abrupt jerking motion to the head and neck and suddenly you have serious neck, shoulder, back pain. Standard X-rays of the neck may not show any injuries.

Sciatica Pain

When your rear or leg muscles worsen when sitting for a long period of time, climbing stairs, walking, or running it might be sciatica.

Arachnoiditis: Spinal Pain

Inflamed tissue, which surrounds the spinal cord caused by injury, infection, or other assaults can cause great disability and pain. Read more.

Phantom Limb Pain

Phantom pain refers to the sensation of pain felt by patients who have had a limb amputated. Treatments are usually disappointing and do not provide relief.

Pelvic Pain Causes and Symptoms

Although pelvic pain often refers to pain in the region of women's internal reproductive organs, pelvic pain can be present in either sex and can stem from multiple causes.

PAIN MEDICATIONS

Over-the-counter (OTC) pain relievers include:
Acetaminophen (Tylenol)

Nonsteroidal anti-inflammatory drugs (NSAIDs), including ibuprofen (Motrin, Advil), naproxen (Aleve, Naprosyn) or diclofinac gel.

Both acetaminophen and NSAIDs reduce fever and relieve pain caused by muscle aches and stiffness, but only NSAIDs can also reduce inflammation (swelling and irritation). Acetaminophen and NSAIDs also work differently. NSAIDs relieve pain by reducing the production of prostaglandins, which are hormone-like substances that cause pain. Acetaminophen works on the parts of the brain that receive the "pain messages." NSAIDs are also available in a prescription strength that can be prescribed by your physician.

Using NSAIDs increase the risk of heart attack or stroke and have also been known to cause stomach ulcers and bleeding. They can also cause kidney problems.

Topical pain relievers are also available without a doctor's prescription. These products include creams, lotions, or sprays that are applied to the skin in order to relieve pain from sore muscles and arthritis. Some examples of topical pain relievers include Aspercreme, BenGay, Icy Hot, and Capzasin-P.

PRESCRIPTION PAIN RELIEVERS

Prescription pain relievers include:
Corticosteroids

Opioids

Antidepressants

Anticonvulsants (anti-seizure medications)

Nonsteroidal anti-inflammatory drugs (NSAIDs)

Lidocaine patches

WHAT ARE CORTICOSTEROIDS?

Prescription corticosteroids provide relief for inflamed areas of the body by easing swelling, redness, itching and allergic reactions. Corticosteroids can be used to treat allergies, asthma and arthritis. When used to control pain, they are generally given in the form of pills or injections that target a certain joint. Examples include: prednisone, prednisolone, and methylprednisolone.

Prescription corticosteroids are strong medicines and may have serious side effects, including:

Weight gain and salt retention

Peptic ulcer disease

Mood changes

Trouble sleeping

Weakened immune system

Thinning of the bones and skin

High sugar levels

To minimize these potential side effects, corticosteroids are prescribed in the lowest dose possible for as short of a length of time as needed to relieve the pain.

WHAT ARE OPIOIDS?

Opioids are narcotic pain medications that contain natural, synthetic or semi-synthetic opiates. Opioids are often used for acute pain, such as short-term pain after surgery. Some examples of opioids include:

Codeine

Fentanyl

Hydrocodone-acetaminophen (Vicodin)

Morphine

Oxycodone

Oxycodone-acetaminophen (Percocet)

Opioids are effective for severe pain and do not cause bleeding in the stomach or other parts of the body, as can some other types of pain relievers.

However, they can be extremely addictive and doctors will try to find alternatives to prescribing them. It is rare for people to become addicted to opioids if the drugs are used to treat pain for a short period of time. But if used to treat chronic pain, the risk of addiction is real and potentially dangerous.

Side effects of opioids may include:
Drowsiness

Nausea

Constipation

Itching

Breathing problems

Addiction

WHAT ARE ANTIDEPRESSANTS?

Antidepressants are drugs that can treat pain and/or emotional conditions by adjusting levels of neurotransmitters (natural chemicals) in the brain. These medications can increase the availability of the body's signals for well-being and relaxation, enabling pain control for some people with chronic pain conditions that do not completely respond to usual treatments. Research suggests certain antidepressants (tricyclics) work best for neuropathic or nerve pain. Chronic pain conditions treated by low-dose antidepressants include some types of headaches (like migraines) and menstrual pain. Some antidepressant medications include:

Selective serotonin reuptake inhibitors (SSRIs) such as citalopram (Celexa), fluoxetine (Prozac), paroxetine (Paxil), and sertraline (Zoloft)

Tricyclic antidepressants such as amitriptyline, desipramine (Norpramin), doxepin (Silenor), imipramine (Tofranil), and nortriptyline (Pamelor)

Serotonin and norepinephrine reuptake inhibitors (SNRIs) such as venlafaxine (Effexor) and duloxetine (Cymbalta)

These drugs require a steady dose of the medicine buildup in the body over a period of time to work. The doses needed to treat pain are often lower than those needed to treat depression.

Generally, SSRIs and SNRIs have fewer side effects than tricyclic antidepressants. The most common side effects with antidepressants include:

Blurry vision

Constipation

Difficulty urinating

Dry mouth

Fatigue

Nausea

Headache

WHAT ARE ANTICONVULSANTS?

Anticonvulsants are drugs typically used to treat seizure disorders. Some of these medications are shown to be effective in treating pain as well. The exact way in which these medicines control pain is unclear but it is thought that they minimize the effects of nerves that cause pain. Some examples include carbamazepine (Tegretol), gabapentin (Neurontin), and pregabalin (Lyrica). In general, anticonvulsants are well tolerated. The most common side effects include:

Drowsiness

Dizziness

Fatigue

Nausea

OTHER PAIN TREATMENTS

Another means of topical pain relief comes in the form of a lidocaine (Lidoderm) patch, which is a prescription medication. If your pain is not relieved by the usual treatments, your doctor may refer you to a pain management specialist. Doctors who specialize in pain management may try other treatments such as certain types of physical therapy or other kinds of medicine. They may also recommend TENS, a procedure that uses patches placed on the skin to send signals that may help stop pain.

Patient-controlled analgesia (PCA) is a method of pain control that allows the patient to control the amount of pain medication administered. This is often used in the hospital to treat pain. By pushing a button on a computerized pump, the patient receives a pre-measured dose of pain medicine. The pump is connected to a small tube that allows medicine to be injected intravenously (into a vein), subcutaneously (just under the skin), or into the spinal area.

WHAT ARE THE TREATMENTS FOR CHRONIC PAIN?

The treatments for chronic pain are as diverse as the causes. From over-the-counter and prescription drugs to mind/body techniques to acupuncture, there are a lot of approaches. But when it comes to treating chronic pain, no single technique is guaranteed to produce complete pain relief. Relief may be found by using a combination of treatment options.

DRUG THERAPY: NONPRESCRIPTION AND PRESCRIPTION

Milder forms of pain may be relieved by over-the-counter medications such as Tylenol (acetaminophen) or nonsteroidal anti-inflammatory drugs (NSAIDs) such as aspirin, ibuprofen, and naproxen. Both acetaminophen and NSAIDs relieve pain caused by muscle aches and stiffness, and additionally NSAIDs reduce inflammation (swelling and irritation). Topical pain relievers are also available, such as creams, lotions, or sprays that are applied to the skin in order to relieve pain and inflammation from sore muscles and arthritis.

If over-the-counter drugs do not provide relief, your doctor may prescribe stronger medications, such as muscle relaxants, anti-anxiety drugs (such as diazepam [Valium]), antidepressants (like duloxetine [Cymbalta] for musculoskeletal pain), prescription NSAIDs such as celecoxib (Celebrex), or a short course of stronger painkillers (such as codeine, fentanyl [Duragesic, Actiq], oxycodone and acetaminophen (Percocet, Roxicet, Tylox) or hydrocodone and acetaminophen (Lorcet, Lortab, and Vicodin). A limited number of steroid injections at the site of a joint problem can reduce swelling and inflammation.

An epidural might be given for spinal stenosis or lower back pain.

In July 2015, the FDA asked that both prescription and over-the-counter NSAIDs strengthen their warning labels to indicate the potential risk of heart attacks and strokes. The risk increases with higher doses of the drugs. In addition, there is also the possibility of developing bleeding stomach ulcers.

Sometimes, a group of nerves that causes pain to a specific organ or body region can be blocked with local medication. The injection of this nerve-numbing substance is called a nerve block. Although many kinds of nerve blocks exist, this treatment cannot always be used. Often blocks are not possible, are too dangerous, or are not the best treatment for the problem. You doctor can advise you as to whether this treatment is appropriate for you. Patient-controlled analgesia (PCA) is another method of pain control. By pushing a button on a computerized pump, the patient is able to self-administer a premeasured dose of pain medicine infused with opiods. The pump is connected to a small tube that allows medicine to be injected intravenously (into a vein), subcutaneously (just under the skin), or into the spinal area. This is often used in the hospital to treat pain in post-traumatic or post-surgical pain as well as terminal cancer pain.

TRIGGER POINT INJECTIONS

Trigger point injection is a procedure used to treat painful areas of muscle that contain trigger points, or knots of muscle that form when muscles do not relax. During this procedure, a healthcare professional, using a small needle, injects a local anesthetic that sometimes includes a steroid into a trigger point (sterile salt water is sometimes injected). With the injection, the trigger point is made inactive and the pain is alleviated. Usually, a brief course of treatment will result in sustained relief.

Trigger point injection is used to treat muscle pain in the arms, legs, lower back, and neck. In addition, this approach has been used to treat fibromyalgia, tension headaches, and myofascial pain syndrome (chronic pain involving tissue that surrounds muscle) that does not respond to other treatment.

Onabotulinumtoxina (Botox) is a toxin that blocks signals from the nerves to the muscles. It can also be injected to alleviate chronic migraine headaches. The procedure involves multiple injections around the head and neck every 12 weeks and may alleviate pain for up to three months.

SURGICAL IMPLANTS

When standard medicines and physical therapy fail to offer adequate pain relief, you may be a candidate for a surgical implant to help you control pain. When they are used, which is rare, there are two main types of implants to control pain:

Intrathecal Drug Delivery. Also called infusion pain pumps or spinal drug delivery systems. The surgeon makes a pocket under the skin that's large enough to hold a medicine pump. The pump is usually about one inch thick and three inches wide. The surgeon also inserts a catheter, which carries pain medicine from the pump to the intrathecal space around the spinal cord. The implants deliver medicines such as morphine or a muscle relaxant directly to the spinal cord, where pain signals travel. For this reason, intrathecal drug delivery can provide significant pain control with a fraction of the dose that would be required with pills. In addition, the system can cause fewer side effects than oral medications because less medicine is required to control pain.

Spinal Cord Stimulation Implants. In spinal cord stimulation, low-level electrical signals are transmitted to the spinal cord or to specific nerves to block pain signals from reaching the brain. This method being especially used for back and limb pain. In this procedure, a device that delivers the electrical signals is surgically implanted in the body. A remote control is used by the patient to turn the current off and on or to adjust the intensity of the signals. Some devices cause what's described as a pleasant, tingling sensation while others do not.

Two kinds of spinal cord stimulation systems are available. The unit that is more commonly used is fully implanted and has a pulse generator and a non-rechargeable battery. The other system includes an antenna, transmitter, and a receiver that relies upon radio frequency. The latter system's antenna and transmitter are carried outside the body, while the receiver is implanted inside the body.

TENS

Transcutaneous electrical nerve stimulation therapy, more commonly referred to as TENS, uses electrical stimulation to diminish pain. During the procedure, low-voltage electrical current is delivered through electrodes that are placed on the skin near the source of pain. The electricity from the electrodes stimulates the nerves in an affected area and sends signals to the brain that "scramble" normal pain signals. TENS is not painful and may be effective therapy to mask pain such as diabetic neuropathy. However, TENS for chronic low back pain is not effective and cannot be recommended, says the American Academy of Neurology (AAN).

BIOELECTRIC THERAPY

Bioelectric therapy relieves pain by blocking pain messages to the brain. Bioelectric therapy also prompts the body to produce chemicals called endorphins (endorphins are also released by exercise) that decrease or eliminate painful sensations by blocking the message of pain from being delivered to the brain. Bioelectric therapy can be used to treat many chronic and acute conditions causing pain, such as back pain, muscle pain, headaches and migraines, arthritis, TMJ disorder, diabetic neuropathy, and scleroderma. Bioelectric therapy is effective in providing temporary pain control, but it should be used as part of a total pain management program. When used along with conventional pain-relieving medications, bioelectric treatment may allow pain sufferers to reduce their dose of some pain relievers by up to 50%.

PHYSICAL THERAPY

Physical therapy helps to relieve pain by using special techniques that improve movement and function impaired by an injury or disability. Along with employing stretching, strengthening, and pain-relieving techniques, a physical therapist may use, among other things, TENS to aid treatment.

EXERCISE

Although resting for short periods can alleviate pain, too much rest may actually increase pain and put you at greater risk of injury when you again attempt movement. Research has shown that regular exercise can diminish pain in the long term by improving muscle tone, strength, and flexibility. Exercise may also cause a release of endorphins, the body's natural painkillers. Some exercises are easier for certain chronic pain sufferers to perform than others; try swimming, biking, walking, rowing, and yoga.

PSYCHOLOGICAL TREATMENT

When you are in pain, you may have feelings of anger, sadness, hopelessness, and/or despair. Pain can alter your personality, disrupt your sleep, and interfere with your work and relationships. In turn, depression and anxiety, lack of sleep, and feelings of stress can all make pain worse. Psychological treatment provides safe, nondrug methods that can treat your pain directly by reducing high levels of physiological stress that often aggravate pain. Psychological treatment also helps improve the indirect consequences of pain by helping you learn how to cope with the many problems associated with pain.

A large part of psychological treatment for pain is education, helping patients acquire skills to manage a very difficult problem.

ALTERNATIVE THERAPIES

In the past decade, many people have found relief for their pain in mind-body therapies, acupuncture, and some nutritional supplements. Others use massage, chiropractic and osteopathic (bone) manipulation therapies, therapeutic touch, certain herbal therapies, and dietary approaches to alleviate pain. However, there is little if any scientific evidence supporting these therapies for pain relief.

MIND-BODY THERAPIES

Mind-body therapies are treatments that are meant to help the mind's ability to affect the functions and symptoms of the body. Mind-body therapies use various approaches including relaxation techniques, meditation, guided imagery, biofeedback, and hypnosis. Relaxation techniques can help alleviate discomfort related to chronic pain. Visualization may be another worthwhile pain-controlling technique. Try the following exercise: Close your eyes and try to call up a visual image of the pain, giving it shape, color, size, motion. Now try slowly altering this image, replacing it with a more harmonious, pleasing and smaller image. Another approach is to keep a diary of your pain episodes and the causative and corrective factors surrounding them. Review your diary regularly to explore avenues of possible change. Strive to view pain as part of life, not all of it.

Electromyographic (EMG) biofeedback may alert you to the ways in which muscle tension is contributing to your pain and help you learn to control it. Hypnotherapy and self-hypnosis may help you block or transform pain through refocusing techniques. One self-hypnosis strategy, known as glove anesthesia, involves putting yourself in a trance, placing a hand over the painful area, imagining that the hand is relaxed, heavy, and numb, and envisioning these sensations as replacing other, painful feelings in the affected area.

Relaxation techniques such as meditation or yoga have been shown to reduce stress-related pain when they are practiced regularly. The gentle stretching of yoga is particularly good for strengthening muscles without putting additional strain on the body.

ACUPUNCTURE

Acupuncture is thought to decrease pain by increasing the release of endorphins, chemicals that block pain. Many acu-points are near nerves. When stimulated, these nerves cause a dull ache or feeling of fullness in the muscle. The stimulated muscle sends a message to the central nervous system (the brain and spinal cord), causing the release of endorphins that block the message of pain from being delivered to the brain. Acupuncture may be useful as an accompanying treatment for many pain-related conditions, including headache, low back pain, menstrual cramps, carpal tunnel syndrome, tennis elbow, fibromyalgia, osteoarthritis (especially of the knee), and myofascial pain. Acupuncture also may be an acceptable alternative to or may be included as part of a comprehensive pain management program.

CHIROPRACTIC TREATMENT AND MASSAGE

Chiropractic treatment is the most common nonsurgical treatment for back pain. Improvements of people undergoing chiropractic manipulations were noted in some trials. However, the treatment's effectiveness in treating chronic back and neck pain has not been supported by compelling evidence from the majority of clinical trials. Further studies are currently assessing the effectiveness of chiropractic care for pain management. Osteopathic doctors, those with a "D.O." after their names, are also trained in bone manipulation techniques similar to that of chiropractors. Massage is being increasingly used by people suffering from pain, mostly to manage chronic back and neck problems. Massage can reduce stress and relieve tension by enhancing blood flow. This treatment also can reduce the presence of substances that may generate and sustain pain. Available data suggest that massage therapy, like chiropractic manipulations, holds considerable promise for managing back pain. However, it is not possible to draw final conclusions regarding the effectiveness of massage to treat pain because of the shortcomings of available studies.

THERAPEUTIC TOUCH AND REIKI HEALING

Therapeutic touch and reiki healing are thought to help activate the self-healing processes of an individual and therefore reduce pain. Although these so-called "energy-based" techniques do not require actual physical contact, they do involve close physical proximity between practitioner and patient. In the past few years, several reviews evaluated published studies on the efficacy of these healing approaches to ease pain and anxiety and improve health. Although several studies showed beneficial effects with no significant adverse side effects, the limitations of some of these studies make it difficult to draw definitive conclusions. Further studies are needed before these approaches for pain treatment can be recommended.

NUTRITIONAL SUPPLEMENTS

Dietary supplements, such as fish oils and SAMe, also show some evidence of benefit, although more research is needed.

HERBAL REMEDIES

It has been difficult to draw conclusions about the effectiveness of herbs, though there are a few, such as white willow bark, devil's claw, cat's claw, ginger, and turmeric, that have some evidence supporting their use. If you decide to use herbal preparations to better manage your pain, tell your doctor: Some herbs may interact with drugs you are receiving for pain or other conditions and may harm your health.

DIETARY APPROACHES TO TREATING PAIN

Some people believe that changing dietary fat intake and/or eating plant foods that contain anti-inflammatory agents can help ease pain by limiting inflammation.

A mostly raw vegetarian diet was found helpful for some people with fibromyalgia, but this study was not methodologically strong. One study of women with premenstrual symptoms suggested that a low-fat vegetarian diet was associated with decreased pain intensity and duration. Weight loss achieved by a combination of dietary changes and increased physical activity has been shown to be helpful for people suffering from osteoarthritis. Still, further research is needed to determine the effectiveness of dietary modifications as a pain treatment.

THINGS TO CONSIDER

Alternative therapies are not always benign. As mentioned, some herbal therapies can interact with other medications you may be taking. Always talk to your doctor before trying an alternative approach and be sure to tell all your doctors what alternative treatments you are using.

Other Options: Pain Clinics

Many people suffering from chronic pain are able to gain some measure of control over it by trying many of the above treatments on their own. But for some, no matter what treatment approach they try, they still suffer from debilitating pain. For them, pain clinics -- special care centers devoted exclusively to dealing with intractable pain may be the answer. Some pain clinics are associated with hospitals and others are private; in either case, both inpatient and outpatient treatment are usually available.

Pain clinics generally employ a multidisciplinary approach, involving physicians, psychologists, and physical therapists. The patient as well should take an active role in his or her own treatment. The aim in many cases is not only to alleviate pain but also to teach the chronic sufferer how to come to terms with pain and function in spite of it.

Various studies have shown as much as 50% improvement in pain reduction for chronic pain sufferers after visiting a pain clinic, and most people learn to cope better and can resume normal activities.

MANAGEMENT OF PAIN WITHOUT MEDICATIONS

What is non-pharmacological pain management?
Non-pharmacological pain management is the management of pain without medications. This method utilizes ways to alter thoughts and focus concentration to better manage and reduce pain. Methods of non-pharmacological pain include:

Education and psychological conditioning

Not knowing what to expect with cancer treatment is very stressful. However, if you are prepared and can anticipate what will happen, your stress level will be much lower. To decrease your anxiety about cancer treatment, consider the following:

Ask for an explanation of each step of a procedure in detail, utilizing simple pictures or diagrams when available.

Meet with the person who will be performing the procedure and write down answers to questions.

Tour the room where the procedure will take place.

Ask what you can expect as an outcome of the treatment.

HYPNOSIS

With hypnosis, a psychologist or doctor guides you into an altered state of consciousness. This helps you to focus or narrow your attention to reduce discomfort. Methods for hypnosis include:

Imagery: Guiding you through imaginary mental images of sights, sounds, tastes, smells, and feelings can help shift attention away from the pain.

Distraction: Distraction is usually used to help children, especially babies. Using colorful, moving objects or singing songs, telling stories, or looking at books or videos can distract preschoolers. Older children and adults find watching TV or listening to music helpful. Use distraction appropriately, and not in place of an explanation of what to expect.

Relaxation/guided imagery: Guiding you through relaxation exercises such as deep breathing and stretching can often reduce discomfort

Other non-pharmacological pain management may utilize alternative therapies such as comfort therapy, physical and occupational therapy, psychosocial therapy/counseling, and neurostimulation to better manage and reduce pain. Examples of these non-pharmacological pain management techniques include the following:

COMFORT THERAPY

Comfort therapy may involve the following:

Companionship

Exercise

Heat/cold application

Lotions/massage therapy

Meditation

Music, art, or drama therapy

Pastoral counseling

Positioning

Physical and occupational therapy

Physical and occupational therapy may involve the following:
Aquatherapy

Tone and strengthening

Desensitization

Psychosocial therapy/counseling

Psychosocial therapy/counseling may involve the following:

Individual counseling

Family counseling

Group counseling

Neurostimulation

Neurostimulation may involve the following:

Transcutaneous electrical nerve stimulation (TENS)

Acupuncture

Acupressure

PAIN CONTROL AFTER SURGERY

The importance of discussing pain control before your surgery

Discuss pain control options with your physician before you have surgery. Talk about pain control methods that have worked well, or not worked well for you in the past. Also, discuss the following with your physician:

Concerns you have about medications

Medications that have not worked well for you

Allergies you have to any medications or drugs

Side effects of pain medications that might occur

Prescription and over-the-counter medications you take for other conditions

The best way of administering pain medication for you

Pain medications are given in one of the following ways:
Upon request - You can ask the nurse for pain medicine as you need it.

Pain pills or shots given at set times - Instead of waiting

until you experience pain, you are given pain medicine at certain, regular times throughout the day to keep the pain under control.

Patient controlled analgesia (called PCA) You control the administration of the pain medicine by pressing a button to inject medicine through an intravenous tube in the vein.

Patient controlled epidural analgesia (called PCEA) This type of administration provides continuous pain relief. A tube is inserted in the spine, and when you press a button, the pain medicine goes into an epidural tube, which is inserted in the back.

Your physicians and nurses will want to know how your pain medicine is working and whether or not you are still experiencing pain. The physician will change the medicine, and/or dosage, if necessary.

PSYCHOLOGICAL THERAPY

Chronic pain can have profound psychological effects, including feelings of hopelessness, anger, sadness, and even despair. These feelings can interfere with your ability to perform your job or your normal daily activities. Psychological therapy can help you to cope with the effects of pain on you and those around you. There are also specific psychological techniques that can actually help to reduce pain.Your treatment plan may include the following psychological therapies:

Individual and group counseling

Biofeedback

Relaxation techniques

Self-hypnosis

Visual imaging

Learning or conditioning techniques

WHAT CAN A PSYCHOLOGIST DO FOR MY PHYSICAL PAIN?

Pain is a "whole person" experience. Most people experience pain physically, emotionally, socially and intellectually. Pain can inhibit a normal productive life: it can limit your ability to concentrate, participate in physical activities and enjoy social interactions. Psychological evaluation and treatment can help many individuals develop specific skills that relieve the suffering of pain and thus increase their quality of life.

WHAT HAPPENS DURING A PSYCHOLOGICAL EVALUATION?

During your psychological evaluation, we hope to gain an understanding of your situation so that we can provide you with some relief from the psychological consequences of your pain. A psychological evaluation is an efficient way of obtaining the necessary personal and historical information to assist you in getting effective medical care and pain relief. As part of the initial consultation, you will be asked to complete several psychological tests and questionnaires. Combined with a personal interview, psychological testing helps you and your physician understand and plan the best possible multidisciplinary treatment. Professional recommendations are normally made after the initial evaluation is completed. We will discuss with you the results of your psychological evaluation and your individualized treatment recommendations prior to your agreement to enter treatment at the Pain Management Center.

WHAT PSYCHOLOGICAL EVALUATION IS NOT?

Some patients are concerned that the psychological evaluation might imply that their pain is imagined rather than felt; this is not the case. In fact, pain that is delusional cannot be alleviated through psychological treatments. Physical pain is normally recognized by the brain and, thus, has many effects on your well-being. It is these effects that we hope to identify during the psychological evaluation.

WHAT PSYCHOLOGICAL TECHNIQUES ARE USED?

Psychological therapy addresses both the physical and the emotional suffering associated with pain. Psychotherapy is offered in both individual and group settings. Specific techniques include:

Biofeedback/Relaxation Training: Many patients benefit from learning how to control their responses to chronic pain. Biofeedback and relaxation training teach you how to release the tension and anxiety that often make painful physical conditions more excruciating.

Behavioral Techniques

Self-Monitoring: Most patients will be asked to keep a diary of their pain, observing how pain levels increase or decrease over time. By monitoring your pain, you can develop an appreciation of your ability to control and manage levels of pain using skills you have learned.

Paced Progressive Increases in Activity Levels: By encouraging the slow and steady introduction of or increase in activity, patients start to feel an improvement in their quality of life. Pain can be very debilitating, but helping patients improve their social, occupational and recreational activity levels can be helpful.

Cognitive Techniques

Self-Hypnosis and Visual Imagery: These techniques help you control pain that interferes with your occupational and sleep patterns. Through self-hypnosis, many patients report reduced levels of pain and an increased ability to concentrate on meaningful pursuits.

Emotional Management: Over time, pain can be very distressing, leading to depression, anxiety and social turmoil. Psychological therapy can assist you in reducing the emotional distress associated with chronic pain. By learning these techniques, your pain can be transformed and your suffering reduced.

HOME TREATMENT AIDS

Office visits also include many helpful self-aid materials that enable patients to maximize the effects of treatment in the shortest time possible. Professional materials instructing you in the self-management approach to chronic pain and professionally produced relaxation and self-hypnosis tapes are provided.

ARE SESSIONS WITH THE PSYCHOLOGIST CONFIDENTIAL?

In almost all situations, you control who access to the information has disclosed during your interview sessions with your psychiatrist. There are some unusual exceptions to this rule, however, and you need to be aware of them. Information regarding child abuse, elder abuse or the need to protect you and others from physical harm or immediate danger must be reported to the appropriate persons by state law.

CONCLUSION

Pain is your body's way of telling you something is wrong. It is normal to expect a certain amount of pain following surgery; however, if pain does not subside with pain medication, there may be a more serious problem. Your physicians and nurses will ask about your pain because they want you to be comfortable. It is important that they be alerted if their efforts to control your pain are not effective. With today's new and improved pain medications, there is no reason for anyone to tolerate severe pain. By effectively treating pain, you will heal faster, have fewer complications following surgery, and be able to go home and resume normal activities sooner.